British Association of Holistic

CN00661295

A Guide to Herbs for Horses

Keith Allison

VETERINARY ADVISER
Christopher Day MRCVS

J. A. Allen
London

Contents

1 History of the use of herbs in medicine

The use of herbs in medicine can be traced back thousands of years. The Chinese Emperor Shennung, who lived around 2700 BC, studied herbs in great detail, and the Shennung herbal, which is believed to be one of the oldest, lists the medical use of around 365 herbal substances. They were grouped into three categories: non-toxic, mildy toxic, and toxic. Amongst these plants were *Ephedra* species, used for bronchial problems, the purgative *Ricinus communis*, and the opium poppy, *Papaver somniferum*. These plants are the basis for the modern medicines ephedrine, castor oil, and morphine respectively.

The Elbers papyrus, which was written about 1500 BC, is perhaps the most famous artefact concerning ancient pharmacy. It is claimed that it was found between the knees of one of the mummies at Thebes. It contained over 800 remedies, involving the use of plants and many other substances such as minerals. As well as their use in the treatment of disease, herbs formed an important part of the diet of the Egyptians and their effects on the body were well known. In common with subsequent generations the Egyptians were fanatically preoccupied with bowel movement, and plants such as rhubarb, castor oil and senna were regularly used as laxatives. Senna was so highly prized that it was reserved for the aristocracy and known as 'guardian of the royal bowel movement'.

The Greek physician Hippocrates (*c.* 460–380 BC), revered by the modern world as the Father of Medicine, described both the beneficial and harmful effects of plants; he also knew that there is a close relationship between nutrition and medicine. Medical practices were based on the philosophy of Hippocrates up to the time of Paracelsus in the sixteenth century.

Probably because herbal medicine has evolved over many centuries and in many cultures, there are a number of different approaches to the subject. This does not mean that there is a right and a wrong approach, only that there are different routes to the same goal.

The difference between modern technological medicines and traditional therapies which make use of natural materials is that modern drugs are normally used to attack the symptom, whereas traditional therapies treat the body itself. Whilst modern drugs may be claimed to have saved thousands of lives, their use must be kept in proper perspective. Medicine alone has never cured anything; it is the body's own healing process which does this.

Medicine of any kind is only successful if it removes the barriers to healing. Modern drugs often have unacceptable side effects, and their manufacture involves the use of animal experimentation, which many find unacceptable when there is a viable alternative.

Up until the first half of the twentieth century the study of pharmacognosy (the study of drugs derived from plants) was part of the education of all medical students and those training as chemists. This fell out of vogue as the twentieth-century sciences developed, promising to be the answer to all the medical problems of both man and beast.

Prior to the 1940s, herbal medications were listed alongside chemical drugs, and even today 50 per cent of the thousands of drugs in common use are either derived from plants or contain chemical imitations of plant compounds. During the rise of the pharmaceutical industry in the 1950s herbal medicine began to be dismissed as outdated. The accumulation of wisdom over thousands of years was effectively debunked overnight by the pharmaceutical industry itself, which suddenly had a pill for everything. Despite the fact that plants were the basis for the majority of the new 'wonder drugs' the idea was successfully propagated that herbal medicine was obsolete. This was done for financial reasons; plants cannot be patented, whereas chemically created molecules can!

At the same time, the idea was also being cultivated that herbal medicines could not be used for 'heroic' measures. Despite the fact that they had been used successfully in this way for thousands of years, the idea gained momentum. Herbal medicine came to be seen as a 'second' or complementary therapy, something to be considered once 'real' medicines had been used (which is one of the reasons for the modern myth that all natural medicines are safe). In fact, there are many instances where horses have been saved from destruction using herbal medicine, when modern technological medicines have failed.

The general use of the word 'herb' covers plant materials with a wide variety of chemical components, offering the potential for a myriad of chemical interactions. They may either be used for gentle nutritional therapy, or for specific medicinal purposes. At one end of the scale are the simple pure herbs such as garlic, and at the other end are those which are very toxic and deadly poisonous either in their own right, or in combination with other substances.

Today there is a swing away from technological medicines towards the use of herbs and other natural therapies. Health food shops are flourishing, and chemist's shelves are stocked with an increasing number of natural remedies. Along with the renewed interest in the subject, and a market for herbal remedies, comes a host of new products to fill the need.

The veterinary market follows closely on the heels of the human market, and there has been an increase in the number of products available for horses which contain herbs. Herbs are included in compound feeds, and many are available as proprietary products sold for a particular purpose. Unfortunately there are pitfalls associated with the use of these products, as we shall see below.

2 Nutrition and medicine: the effect of herbs on the body

It can be clearly demonstrated that there is no difference between nutrition and medicine. In the words of Hippocrates, 'let food be thy medicine, and medicine thy food'. Anything taken by mouth has an effect on the body. Obviously the effect depends on the substance and its concentration.

The entire spectrum of available food must be taken into the equation, as each component has both an individual and a combined effect. In nature, the horse knows this by instinct and will select specific foods in order to maintain optimum nutrition. The domesticated horse has no choice and must eat what he is given, which places this heavy responsibility on the owner.

Whilst all plants have an effect on the body, herbal medicine is mainly concerned with the study of those which may be used for therapeutic purposes. Most herbs have several properties and the most dominant one usually determines the species to be used. There are two main types of medicinal substances found in herbs, and they are complementary to each other, which is the reason that herbs must be used whole. The two substances are the primary healing agents, which many modern technological medicines are based on; and the secondary compounds, which ensure that the body is receptive to the primary agent. Secondary agents also buffer and moderate the effect of the primary agent.

The active constituents of herbs

Alkaloids

Alkaloids are one of the most common ingredients in plants, and they have varying toxic or medical effects on the body. They can be stimulants, depressives, narcotics, or painkillers. Alkaloids are the basis for many modern drugs, such as morphine, quinine, atropine and codeine. They exist in small quantities in many plant species and can act as catalysts to healing agents in others. Many narcotic drugs are composed of alkaloids; apart from the commonly known ones, such as marihuana from hemp and opium from the poppy, they occur in many other plant materials. Nutmeg, for example, contains a powerful narcotic called myristicin.

Bitters

Bitters are bitter to the taste, hence the name. They are used for relieving digestive disorders and to stimulate the appetite. They increase the flow of gastric juices and excite the nerves which regulate the muscular movements of the digestive tract. Many bitter drugs, otherwise known as bitter tonics, are effective in the horse; but a large number of remedies are required because what suits one horse may not suit another. They are especially useful for digestive upsets which may be caused by the ingredients of modern compound feeds. Bitter drugs include gentian, calumba, and cinchona among many others. Bitters also have other properties, some being sedative, others antimicrobial.

Flavonoids and bioflavonoids

Most herbs containing flavonoids are diuretic, some are antispasmodic, and others are anti-inflammatory. Bioflavonoids are known to strengthen the body's capillaries, and are useful to treat conditions which arise as a result of vulnerable tissue.

Glycosides

Glycosides are compounds of glucose and other substances. The cardiac glycosides, such as digoxin and digitoxin, from the foxglove, are traditionally used in the treatment of heart failure. These must be used with extreme caution under veterinary guidance only. Some glycosides form foam when mixed with water and are highly toxic (see saponins).

Mucilage

Mucilaginous substances are contained in plants such as comfrey, flax and psyllium seeds, as well as in herbs like marshmallow and slippery elm. When mucilage is dissolved in water or body fluids, it forms a sticky viscous gel. This may be used to soothe inflamed and irritated tissue, whilst protecting the surface of the membranes. Mucilage is also used as a mild laxative, as it absorbs water into the bowel which bulks out and loosens the faecal contents.

Saponins

Saponins form a lather (sapo means soap) when they are mixed with water, and they emulsify oils. Some are diuretic, others are expectorant, most are highly toxic. One of their actions is that they cause red blood cells to disintegrate, so they should never be used on broken skin. The saponin in liquorice root has similarities in action to the hormone cortisone which is used in conventional drug therapy to treat inflammation.

Tannins

Tannins have a mainly astringent action. They have the effect of shrinking cells by precipitating proteins from their surface. Astringents may be used internally or externally, and are often used in lotions to harden and protect the skin. They are also capable of stopping external bleeding, and can be used in the treatment of other conditions where the loss of body fluids should be controlled. Astringents which were often used in the treatment of horses include nut-galls, oak bark, and catechu.

Poisons which occur in herbs and other natural substances

Many species of plants contain substances known as toxins, most of which may belong to the above classification, but all of which have the potential to harm the body (the ancient Greek word 'toxicon' meant 'poison for arrows'). Toxicology is a very complex subject, knowledge of which is becoming increasingly important because of the unnatural diet of the modern horse.

The principles of toxicology are relevant to two main areas: first, in relation to the substances available to the horse when grazing, and secondly with regard to the use of feed additives (both synthetic and natural) in feeds and feed supplements.

Toxins are harmful to the body because they are capable of irritating, damaging, or impairing the activity of tissue. Such harm can be the direct result of a single substance, or of a combination of substances producing a poisonous effect.

Substances regarded as poisonous for one species may not be so for another. This is known as 'species difference'. Potentially toxic substances are contained in a great many species of plants, apart from those officially listed as poisons. Under normal circumstances, minor toxins can be ignored reasonably safely. However, knowledge of toxicology is obviously very important in herbal medicine and certain aspects of nutrition (see pp. 12–13).

Biochemically, plants may be grouped according to their toxic principles. There is a vast range of compounds within these groups, many of which, such as alkaloids, can also be used as medicines. In some cases, plants will vary in their toxicity depending on several factors, such as the time of year, and perhaps the time of day. For example, at nine o'clock in the morning the opium poppy is reputed to contain four times as much morphine as it does at twelve noon.

The effects of some listed poisons (together with many other substances) on certain animals can vary greatly. For example, pigs thrive on amounts of acorns which cause poisoning in cattle. Deer are reported to be able to feed on yew and rhododendron, and grey squirrels on *Amanita* mushrooms, all of which may be fatal in other species. There are also variations within certain species: for example, some types of rabbit are not adversely affected by deadly nightshade. Goats are less affected by this plant than many other animals. In some cases the difference may be in part attributed to the basic anatomy of the animal; for example, those with large forestomachs (ruminants) may be able to dilute some toxic substances, or it is broken down before reaching the blood stream. In others there are complex chemical factors involved.

Poisoning can also be a question of degree, depending on the severity of toxicity which has been caused. Sometimes, the effect may be so slight as to go unnoticed. Often problems such as nonspecific allergies, weight loss, lethargy, and mild digestive problems may not necessarily be thought to be associated with toxins, particularly if they are relatively mild. The correct diagnosis may therefore be missed.

It is thought that many horses along with other grazing animals commonly suffer from the effects of mild toxicity. This may be because they are forced to feed on certain plants in the absence of more suitable species. Compound feeds containing unsuitable ingredients, such as by-products from other food manufacturing industries and molasses, probably contribute to the problem, along with the indiscriminate use of synthetic additives and unsuitable herbal supplements.

The reason that feral horses do not normally poison themselves with plants is probably because they have access to an abundance of natural food. Horse-sick, weed-infested pastures present the greatest risk to the modern horse. Some poisonous plants such as bracken and ragwort build up slowly in the system and cause a gradual decline in health as toxins accumulate; others such as a yew can kill a horse immediately. A horse will rarely eat ragwort unless it is broken down and wilted.

Plants found in the United Kingdom which are regarded as potentially poisonous in their own right are alder, black bryony, black nightshade, bracken, buckthorn, celandine, chickweed, columbine, cowbane, darnel, deadly nightshade, flax, foxglove, fritillary, greater corncockle, hellebore, hemp, henbane, herb paris, horsetails, irises, laburnum, larkspur, lily of the valley, lupins, meadow saffron, monks-hood, pimpernels, poppies, potato, privet, ragwort, rhododendron, sandwort, soapwort, sowbread, St John's wort, thornapple, white bryony, and yew.

A plant may poison directly, as a result of chemical action within the tissues, or indirectly by impeding metabolism of vital body substances. An example of indirect poisoning is bracken, which damages thiamine.

The most common causes of fatal or serious poisoning in horses are ragwort, yew, laburnam and bracken. Problems which arise from other plants will vary from a slight stomach upset to more severe problems, depending on a number of other factors.

3 Preparation of herbs

As a herbivore the horse is designed to assimilate the constituents of herbs in their natural state. Properly dried herbs will keep well in a cool dark place, although they are probably best used promptly. Combinations of medicinal herbs may be unpalatable to the horse, and traditionally they were mixed into 'horse balls' with butter or a similar substance. These were then administered either by hand or by using a special instrument to deposit the ball into the back of the mouth, which the horse found difficult to refuse.

Infusions

Infusions are made by using the soft parts of the plants – the stems, flowers and leaves. Boiling water is poured over the herbs and they are left to infuse until cold. Many remedies may be given this way, provided they are palatable. Hay tea is a traditional remedy for invalid horses as is linseed tea, which is a weak version of linseed mash.

Inhalations

The constituents of some herbs may be administered through the respiratory system. The vapours of infusions or decoctions of herbs may be inhaled.

Decoctions

In order to prepare a liquor for oral administration, the harder woody parts of some plants need special treatment if they are to impart their constituents to water. They are usually crushed or ground and boiled vigorously before being allowed to cool for the horse to drink.

Tinctures

The relevant components of a herb required for oral administration may be extracted using a combination of water and alcohol. In this form they may be stored for two years or more, the alcohol acting as a preservative.

4 The diet of the modern horse

The horse has evolved to live on multi-species herbage. His ancestor, Eohippus, which lived on earth 55 million years ago, lived on marshy ground and ate soft succulent fruits, berries and herbage. As the horse evolved it gradually moved further out into more open country, and its diet became a variety of high fibre plains grasses and herbage.

Up until the end of the nineteenth century the horse still had access to a large variety of herbage in pasture and in hay. This, together with simple foods such as oats to provide more energy when required for work, formed the staple diet of most horses. There was nothing complicated about it and horses provided power for work, recreation and war on this diet for generations.

When the horse was ailing there was a host of herbal 'remedies' available, some of which were certainly effective. Others were probably useless or dangerous; there is little doubt that many horses would have died, or been made worse, because of the application of some of the 'remedies' of the time. These concoctions had very little to do with scientific principles, often being formulated by those with no proper training or qualification, sometimes referred to as quacks.

The basic diet of the horse has deteriorated during the twentieth century in two ways. First, as a result of more intensive farming methods, the number of herb species began to decline; today there are only around one quarter of the former species growing in pasture. Secondly, the feed industry began to offer compound feeds containing by-products, and other inappropriate materials such as synthetic vitamins and molasses, which the horse has not even evolved to eat.

Modern equine nutrition is developed from cattle science, which concentrates on converting food to meat or milk in the most cost-efficient way. This approach is basically and seriously flawed because of 'species difference'. The cow is a ruminant, the horse is not. The horse is a physical performer, the cow is not. Also the horse lives to a far greater age than most cows, and therefore potential problems have more time to show than in cattle. Because the horse food industry developed out of the agricultural industry, which made extensive use of by-products, it came to rely on the principles of fortification, using synthetic products. Manufacturing standards were adopted which relied on chemical analysis, rather than on trying to achieve optimum nutrition by using materials which the horse has evolved to eat. Most modern compounded feeds are formulated according to the theories of comparatively narrow scientific disciplines, which apart from being complicated are often blinkered. They take little or no account of botany, herbal science, veterinary medicine, or holism.

Today, unless holistic compound feeds are being given (see pp. 15–16), most horses fed on a combination of grass and forage plus ordinary compound feeds almost certainly have nutritional imbalances. These are caused by a deficiency of the right types of food and an excess of the wrong types. The growth in the market for supplements shows that the horse owner recognises this. There is a host of products available which claim to improve coat and skin, hooves, blood, temperament, and many other problems which would probably not arise if the horse was given a proper diet in the first place. To make matters worse, many of these supplements are formulated according to the same inappropriate science as the feeding stuffs, and many are synthetic or contain unsuitable raw materials such as animal or fish products. Despite concern being expressed about the use of animal and fish products for horses, such things as liver extract and animal fats continue to be used. Inappropriate herbal supplements also abound.

Synthetic vitamins are used by horse owners (and many manufacturers) at a rate which is not scientifically justifiable. Many people do not even realise that they are using them. Apart from their possible effects on the immune system, synthetic vitamins are not absorbed in the same way as natural ones, and their long-term safety in horses has not been tested. Information from many respected scientific institutions shows that very little is known about the requirements, or safe levels, for synthetic vitamins in the equine. It is quite possible that many horses are consuming them at potentially toxic levels in the form of multi-vitamin supplements. Furthermore, their manufacture may depend upon genetic engineering and animal experimentation. The British Association of Holistic Nutrition and Medicine (BAHNM) gives technical advice on these issues and offers general information on the formulation of specific types of products (see p. 41).

The horse owner is becoming increasingly aware of these issues, and there is a growing demand for products which are more compatible with the evolved physiology of the horse. There is an increasing use of products which claim to be natural and generally there is a swing away from anything which is synthetic. There has been a remarkable growth in the use of herbs in equine products (see next chapter), together with an increase in the sales of holistic feeding stuffs and supplements (see p. 41).

5 Guide to feeding stuffs and supplements containing herbs

Herbs are used in both feeding stuffs and supplements. The following is a general guide to their use in these products. They may be conveniently separated into the following groups.

1. Holistic compound feeding stuffs
2. Compound feeding stuffs
3. Forage
4. Pure herbs
5. Proprietary herbal mixtures

Holistic compound feeds

The BAHNM licences holistic compound feeds. They can be identified by a symbol which is displayed on all packaging. The licensing system is administered by the BAHNM in parallel with government departments responsible for associated statutory legislation, such as the Feeding Stuffs Regulations, the Medicine Acts, and the Trade Descriptions Acts.

Holistic products are formulated according to the scientific principles of holism first published by Jan Christian Smuts (1870–1950). It means that all ingredients are in holistic balance with each other, as in nature. They contain no by-products, no artificial products such as synthetic vitamins, no added molasses or syrups, and no animal or fish products.

Many holistic compound feeds may be used for nutritional therapy. They are useful where diet is important in the management of diseases such as laminitis and respiratory problems. Typically they contain up to thirty or more raw materials (including a substantial number of herbs), whereas other modern compounded feeds contain around half that number, some of which may be incompatible with holistic nutrition.

Regulatory information

The exact nature and inclusion rate of every ingredient must be declared. Raw materials, formulations, and manufacture must comply with common 'Quality Standards for Holistic Products'. BAHNM Protocols must be observed at all stages of manufacture to ensure proper standards of safety, quality, efficacy and nutritional viability of the product.

Compound feeds

The majority of ordinary compound feeds contain molasses and artificial products such as synthetic vitamins. They may also contain any number of the 140 or so ingredients available to the feed industry from many sources worldwide. Most of these are denatured by-products, and many animal products are listed. By-products of the food industry such as wheat feed and oat feed are commonly used.

Because many of these raw materials are unappetising, it has been common practice for several years to add molasses; there is also an increasing use of the fragrant herbs, such as mint, for the same reason. Some feeds claim to contain effective therapeutic herbage. The inappropriate formulation of such feeds means that they will probably have little or no effect on the physiology of the body (see previous section and p. 22). Most compounded feeds also contain added anti-oxidant chemicals, whose full effects on the body have not been established. These are put in to prevent bacterial degradation of the food in the bag – but as the horse depends on bacteria to digest his food, is this wise?

Regulatory information

The main legislation concerning horse feeds is the Feeding Stuffs Regulations. Under their provisions, ingredients may be declared in a way which does not indicate their true nature, and there is no guaranteed access to specific information concerning any raw materials, including herbs. Most manufacturers are helpful when questioned about their products, but some are not. Commercial expediency is the stated reason for not declaring the ingredients, but without full information the horse owner or veterinarian cannot decide if a food is safe or suitable. The BAHNM helpline will give free information on raw materials used in feeding stuffs and associated matters (see p. 41).

Forage

The evolved physiology of the horse is designed to gain maximum benefit from the nutrients it receives from forage, yet the quality of this part of the diet is often not given proper consideration. As we have seen there is a lack of variety of herbage in most pastures, which of course is reflected in the quality of most forage. Furthermore, fertilising of pasture, while increasing growth, alters the nutritional profile out of all recognition. Ways to improve forage by oversowing with different species of herbage are suggested in Chapter 6. Holistic forage products are also available which provide a nutritional profile reflecting that of traditional meadow.

Manufacturers of some forage products, such as molassed chaff, are introducing a low level of fragrant herbs, such as mint, which probably does not contribute anything positive from a physiological standpoint. However, the horse may enjoy it and this may be good enough.

Regulatory information

The main legislation for forage is the Feeding Stuffs Regulations. Generally there is no requirement to declare the exact nature of added herbs.

Pure herbs

Many pure single herbs are available, most of which are imported and of variable quality. The general quality will be apparent from the appearance and fragrance. Many species are available, but unless the horse owner has appropriate knowledge none of them should be used without specialist independent advice. While some herbs like garlic may be used on a regular basis, those which have the potential for more specific actions should not be used regularly. On no account should they be used to try and effect a cure without properly experienced veterinary advice.

Regulatory information

The main legislation for these products is the Feeding Stuffs Regulations. The manufacturer usually states the nature of the product, for example 'garlic', and it should be clear from the labelling if anything else has been added. There is often a reference on the packaging to the traditional use of such products, or to feeding rates. This can only be regarded as anecdotal information, often inappropriate and unreliable, derived from literature relating to the use of herbs in human medicine. The responsibility for safe and proper use of the product rests with the consumer.

Proprietary herbal mixtures

Mixtures of therapeutic herbage are sold for a specific physiological purpose. These products contain many pitfalls for the unwary, mainly associated with safety, quality and efficacy. Unfortunately most of them are formulated by those with either no proper training or inappropriate qualifications, using information gleaned from human herbals; this approach is scientifically flawed and can be dangerous in some circumstances. For example, a plant as seemingly innocuous as clover has a very different effect in the horse than in the human, owing to differences in the digestive system. Many products contain dubious concoctions of therapeutic herbs such as sedatives, analgesics, and others which should not be used on a regular basis without veterinary advice.

In addition, quality standards are notoriously difficult to maintain. Even if human-quality herbs are used, and very often this is not the case, there can be risks regarding the large amounts of imported products used. Some have contained unidentified toxic substances, and there are increasing concerns in this area. The poisons unit at Guys Hospital, London, has over the past few years received almost 6000 enquiries concerning the possible side effects of alternative remedies and food additives used by humans. Although most were less serious, symptoms of actual poisoning were reported in about 10 per cent of these cases.

Most proprietary herbal products do not declare the exact nature of their ingredients and there is no guaranteed way of finding out what they are. Commercial interests in this market are in danger of overshadowing both wisdom and animal welfare. Apart from the issues above, if veterinary attention is required, the ingredients of any product the horse has been administered cannot be properly taken into consideration when making clinical judgements, since full information is lacking. In addition, if substances have been used which have had the effect of desensitising the body over a period of time, stronger measures may have to be resorted to than would otherwise have been necessary to effect a cure. The reader is warned that this area is a minefield and extreme caution is advised.

Regulatory information

The regulatory legislation concerning herbal mixtures is complex and beyond the scope of this guide. In general terms, such products should only be used if:

> the product has a licence under the Veterinary Medicines Act; or
> the product is licensed under the BAHNM regulations; or
> the exact formulation is known and properly evaluated.

Responsibility for the safe and proper use of unlicensed products rests with the consumer. The BAHNM and other bodies (pp. 41, 47) will provide free help and guidance in these circumstances.

6 Complementary herbage for pastures

As we have seen the ecological changes which have taken place as a result of modern farming methods have drastically reduced the species of herbage available to the modern horse.

Whilst it would be very difficult to re-create the healthier pastures of, say, the mid-nineteenth century, certain species of herbs may be oversown into existing grazing in order to help counteract the imbalance. Unless holistic feeds are being given, other herbage would have to be provided from an external source. If herbal supplements are being used, care must be taken to feed the right species in the correct amounts. Commercially oriented advice must be accepted with caution.

A good basic horse paddock mixture is:

Two varieties of perennial ryegrass (*Lolium perenne*): 50 per cent.
Two varieties of creeping red fescue (*Festuca rubra*): 25 per cent.
Crested dog's tail (*Cynosurus cristatus*): 10 per cent.
Rough or smooth stalked meadow grass (*Poa trivialis* or *Poa pratensis*): 10 per cent.
Wild white clover (*Trifolium repens*): 5 per cent.

Other species such as timothy or cocksfoot may also be used. Dandelion, daisy, nettle, chicory, yarrow, and burnet are also suitable herbs for pastures and are of potential benefit to the grazing horse.

Many others may be considered but the type and quality of the soil affects the way in which various species will grow. The local office of ADAS (Food, Farming, Land and Leisure) is a source of information on local soil conditions and associated subjects.

A comparison between physiologically active components in traditional and modern grasslands

The table below demonstrates the number of species with physiologically active components in two types of grassland. One is a traditional meadow containing 60 species, and one is a modern meadow containing 7 species. The numbers represent the number of species which contained the relevant components. The table is simplistic in that the components have been classified into main groups. There are also many sub-groups, each member of which may demonstrate a different property. Alkaloids, for example, are a very varying and diverse group, some of which are poisons.

The potential for the benefits to health is directly related to the range of components present, and deficiencies may be linked to the onset of disease.

Component	Traditional meadow	Modern meadow
Alkaloids	11	0
Glycosides	6	1
Essential oils	8	0
Tannins	8	1
Saponins	2	0
Pectins	1	0
Amara	3	0
Other specific	14	1
Phytoncides	10	1
Homoeopathic	39	0

7 The use of herbs in optimum nutrition, nutritional therapy and medicine

Optimum nutrition

Optimum nutrition is the goal. It means providing a diet which is closest to the horse's evolved nutritional requirements. By this means, natural good health and vitality can prevail. If optimum nutrition is provided, the need for nutritional therapy and, more especially, medicine will be eliminated or greatly reduced. The best way to achieve this is first and foremost by appropriate healthy grazing and forage, supported with appropriate holistic feeding stuffs and forage products, where required (p. 41).

Nutritional therapy

Nutritional therapy is the use of a herb, or a specific combination of herbs or other plant material, to produce a gentle therapeutic action. It is effective in situations where diet is particularly important in the management of various ailments, such as laminitis. This should not be seen as 'supplementation'; the aim is to change subtly the overall profile of the diet in order to have the desired effect. All ingredients must be synchronised as part of the entire nutritional profile. Discussing individual components or supplements in isolation is an unwise and dangerous practice.

Most compound feeding stuffs do not provide a good base for nutritional therapy, because of the inappropriate raw materials they contain. Treatment which relies on complex and delicate synergies will not be effective when the basic feed ration contains ingredients such as artificial vitamins, high levels of sugars, and possibly anti-oxidant chemicals. Holistic feeds, on the other hand, should be ideal to use as a base feed, where necessary, for nutritional therapy.

Medicine

Plant materials may also be used for a more specific effect on the body. The action of the medicine depends both on the species used and the formulation. Some are complex remedies involving many different ingredients, others are relatively simple. Many drugs which may be used for heroic medicine, such as narcotics, come into this category.

8 Herbs and other plant materials traditionally used for horses and their actions

The physiological effect of many plant materials depends as much on their combined action as upon their individual chemistry. For example, within a single prescription, two or more herbs may display apparently contradictory functions. Often the introduction of a seemingly innocuous herb can trigger a chemical action which could not happen without it, and the effect can be quite dramatic.

It must be emphasised that the information given in this guide should not be regarded as an encouragement to the horse owner to diagnose or treat any disease or condition. That is not to say that valuable herbs such as garlic may not be given in sensible amounts on a regular basis; rather that the chemical properties of any single herb or herbal mixture should be properly evaluated by a suitably qualified person. If in doubt, the horse owner should err on the side of caution and take independent advice (see pp. 41, 47). It should be added that pregnant mares should never be given herbs unless they have been professionally cleared as safe. There are many examples of tragedies occurring in this area.

The wide-ranging list below is representative of herbs and plant materials which were well established in equine veterinary medicine and nutritional therapy before the rise of the pharmaceutical industry. Many are listed poisons, others may produce toxic or other inappropriate results either singly or in combination. It is beyond the scope of this short guide to describe anything other than the basic properties of the species mentioned; the subject should be approached with extreme caution.

Aconite (*Aconitum napellus*)
Constituents: Aconitine, alkaloids
Also known as monkshood and wolfsbane, aconite is

extremely toxic. The medicinal dose is very close to the amount which will poison. The alkaloids act to reduce nerve activity drastically, and also to stimulate the heart and circulation. In minute doses it has been used traditionally as an anodyne and circulatory stimulant. It is safe when given homoeopathically, in the extreme dilutions common to that system of medicine.

Aloe (*Aloe vera*)
Constituents: Glycosides, aloe-emodin, resin

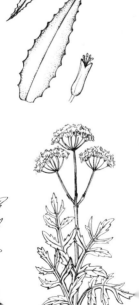

Both the juice and the gel obtained from the plant have medicinal uses. The juice is a powerful purgative, useful in constipation and in colic. It acts by irritating the gut, and is used in conjunction with carminatives. The gel is particularly valuable as a healing agent; it may be applied directly to burns, cuts and wounds. Commercially produced gels are unreliable because of the solvents used in their extraction, and because of their variable contents even some of the so-called 'pure' preparations are so dilute or degenerate as to be ineffective. There is renewed interest in *Aloe vera* preparations and the BAHNM is evaluating the various products available.

Anise (*Pimpinella anisum*)
Constituents: Volatile oil, coumarins, glycosides

The parts of this plant normally used are the seeds. Aniseed assists digestion, and it is useful in the treatment of respiratory problems. When given with saline and other purgatives it can be used to prevent griping; and in conjunction with ginger it assists expulsion of gas from the stomach and bowels.

Arnica (*Arnica montana*)
Constituents: Volatile oil, resins, carotenoids, flavonoids

Arnica is a well-known homoeopathic and herbal treatment for wounds, bruises and many other kinds of injury. When used externally it is applied as ointments or creams; in some circumstances it can cause skin irritation. When used internally it is toxic, except in prepared homoeopathic doses which are best given under the direction of a veterinary surgeon.

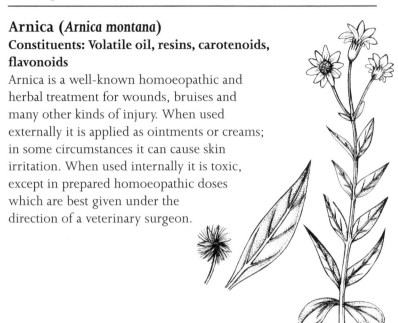

Asafoetida (*Ferula asa-foetida*)
Constituents: Resin, volatile oil, gum

Also known as devil's dung, it is an effective expectorant and traditionally used in the treatment of chronic bronchitis. It is a circulatory stimulant and can also be used to calm intestinal and digestive upsets.

Belladonna (*Atropa belladonna*)
Constituents: Alkaloids

Belladonna depresses the central nervous system and can be deadly if not used appropriately, as its common name, deadly nightshade, suggests. It is effective in reducing spasm in the gut wall, gall bladder and urinary tract, and it can reduce excessive perspiration and salivation. A few drops of the juice in the eye dilates the pupil, which made it popular to facilitate eye examination. Interestingly, Renaissance ladies were in the habit of using it to produce the same effect, in order to make their eyes more attractive – hence the name (Italian, beautiful woman). In homoeopathic medicine it can prove very safe and valuable.

Calabar bean (*Physostigma venenosa*)
Constituents: Physostigmine

A powerful sedative having a profound effect on the spinal column. It paralyses voluntary muscles and reduces skin sensitivity. Traditionally used in horses to control the spasms of tetanus; also in ophthalmic procedures, where it has the effect of dilating the pupil (*see* belladonna). It has also been used to remove the offending matter in cases of impaction of the bowel, amongst other things. Its use can be dangerous.

Calumba (*Jateorhiza palmata*)
Constituents: Alkaloids, bitter glycosides, volatile oil

One of the most valuable bitter tonics, also having a carminative action on the gut, it is more likely to be refused in food than other bitters. Traditionally used with *Nux vomica* and mineral acids in the form of an infusion; or with bicarbonate of soda to treat acid forms of stomach trouble, for example those resulting from carbohydrate fermentations associated with the use of concentrate feeds.

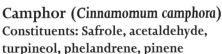

Camphor (*Cinnamomum camphora*)
Constituents: Safrole, acetaldehyde, turpineol, phelandrene, pinene

Applied externally with other agents for the relief of rheumatic pains, and useful for the treatment of sprained tendons, ligaments, and joints. Extensively used in traditional veterinary medicine, both externally, and internally to arrest catarrh and coughs, to check diarrhoea, and to relieve wind in the gut. It is a powerful stimulant in case of collapse, but is damaging to homoeopathic medicines.

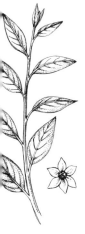

Cannabis
See Indian Hemp

Catechu (*Acacia catechu*)
Constituents: Tannins, flavonoids
Extracted from the heartwood of a tree in the Acacia family. A powerful stringent used in the treatment of diarrhoea, gut infections and irritations. Traditionally combined with opium and chalk to moderate and complement its actions.

Chamomile (*Matricaria chamomilla*)
Constituents: Volatile oils, bisabolol, farnesine, sesquiterpene lactones, cyanogenic glycosides
Also known as German chamomile, this widely used plant is valuable for its calming properties. It relaxes the viscera and is also a valuable bitter tonic useful in remedies for its digestive disorders. In addition, it has anodyne properties and is a valuable homoeopathic remedy.

Cinchona (*Cinchona succirubra*)
Constituents: Alkaloids, glycosides, quinic acid, tannins, cinchona

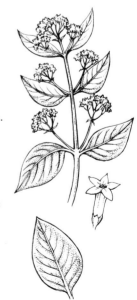

Also known as Jesuit's bark and fever tree. The bark of this tree is the source of quinine. There are several varieties of the tree, some of which are richer in the alkaloids than others. Quinine is probably best known for its use in human medicine against malaria. It has many uses in equine medicine; for the treatment of fever in general and as a bitter digestive tonic. Once used extensively with alcohol in the treatment of equine flu. Should not be used during pregnancy It is safe in homoeopathic form.

Cleavers (*Galium aparine*)
Constituents: Coumarins, tannins, citric acid
Also known as 'goose grass' or 'sticky willie' because of its tiny hooks which seem to attach themselves to everything. It is a reliable diuretic and can be used to treat urinary stones and urinary infections. It stimulates the lymphatic system and is used to cleanse the blood of impurities.

Cocaine (*Erythroxylon coca*)
Constituents: Alkaloids
Traditionally used as a local anaesthetic, most often for allowing surgical procedures to be carried out without pain. Its use internally could contravene the rules of competition sport.

Comfrey (*Symphytum officinale*)
Constituents: Alkaloids, allantoin, tannins, resin, steroidal saponins, pyrrolizidine

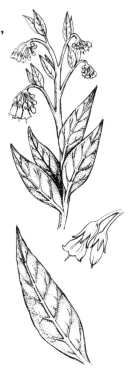

Comfrey has been used for generations to soothe and heal skin wounds. It is rich in calcium and mucilaginous substances, and also contains allantoin which helps cell regeneration. It can be used internally as an astringent in the treatment of diarrhoea and to stop bleeding; it also helps fractured bones to heal, giving rise to its common name of 'knitbone'. Some varieties of comfrey contain pyrrolizidine alkaloids, which have been linked to the formation of tumours when ingested in large amounts over long periods. It is a common ingredient of many proprietary herbal supplements, so care should be exercised. In homoeopathic form it is safe. Other names: knitbone, boneset, blackwort, bruisewort.

Dandelion (Taraxacum officinale)

Constituents: Taraxacin, triterpenes, glycosides, potassium, iron, sterols

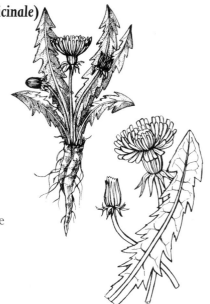

The common name 'pee in the bed' is consistent with its powerful diuretic properties. It is known to be as powerful as synthetic diuretics, but without the side effects. It is used as an aid to cleansing the blood of impurities, as a mild laxative and as a valuable bitter tonic.

Deadly nightshade

See Belladonna

Devil's claw (Harpagophytum procumbens)

Constituents: Iridoid glycosides, beta sitosterols

Devil's claw is primarily used as an inflammation and pain reliever. It can be used in combination with other herbs for the medical relief of arthritis and rheumatism. It takes its name from the shape of the root. The physiological action of devil's claw has been compared to the powerful modern synthetic drugs, cortisone and phenylbutazone. It should not be used in some circumstances, and may not be safe in pregnancy. Its use may contravene competition rules, which means that careful selection of herbal supplements is required, as many contain it.

Digitalis

See Foxglove

Echinacea (*Echinacea angustifolia*)
Constituents: Essential oil, glycoside, polysaccharide, sesquiterpene

Used as a blood cleanser to aid healing, particularly where impure blood is associated with skin problems. It is antibiotic and used to treat wounds, where it reduces putrification and pain. It also may be used to enhance the immune system by stimulating the production of white blood cells. The polysaccharide has an antiviral activity.

Ergot (*Claviceps*)
Constituents: Alkaloids

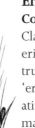

Claviceps is a kind of fungus that infects with varying severity many species of cereal crops. They can be seen protruding from infected seedheads as hard masses called 'ergots'. The ergots are poisonous and although seen relatively infrequently today, they were formerly seen in many crops of rye. Ergot of Rye was used in traditional medicine to constrict the small blood vessels, and was given to mares after parturition, and for inflammation of the coverings of the brain and spinal column. It is not safe to use in pregnancy, and is a dangerous substance to use without proper professional guidance.

Fenugreek (*Trigonella foenum-graecum*)
Constituents: Alkaloid, bitter principle, steroidal saponin, mucilage

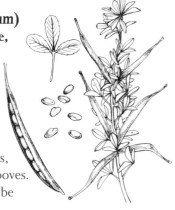

Fenugreek has been used for generations as a fodder crop. Its use in nutrition and medicine dates back to the time of the ancient Egyptians and Hippocrates. It may be given to healthy horses as a conditioner on a regular basis, being good for weight gain, coat and hooves. As it is a uterine stimulant it should not be given to pregnant mares: however, it can be given to the nursing mare to promote milk flow.

Foxglove (*Digitalis purpurea / lanata*)
Constituents: Glycosides, digitoxin, gitoxin, gitaloxin
The leaves of the purple foxglove are the source of digitalis. When dried and finely powdered it can be made into an infusion which affects the heart. It increases the force of the heart beat whilst lessening the frequency of beats. It can also be used to excite the kidneys to produce more urine than usual. Poisonous doses cause the heart to spasm, and death is caused by cardiac paralysis. It is therefore a potentially very dangerous herb.

Garlic (*Allium sativum*)
Constituents: Volatile oil, glucokinins
Garlic is one of the most widely used herbs, and has been used since ancient times. It may be fed regularly to healthy horses as a pure herb. It has a wide spectrum of beneficial effects on the body. It is a good digestive aid, and a good 'warming' remedy for use during the winter. It is used medically in combination with other herbs as an effective antibiotic, antiparasitic, expectorant, and antihistamine.

Gentian (*Gentiana lutea*)
Constituents: Bitter glycosides, alkaloids, flavonoids
Gentian is a pronounced bitter digestive stimulant, containing one of the most bitter substances known, the glycoside amarogentin. It is also an anti-inflammatory. Despite its bitter taste

it will be readily taken by most horses when ground and put into the food. Traditionally used as a general tonic for horses in combination with various other substances. It increases the appetite by stimulating the flow of bile and the digestive juices. It is also used to treat gastrointestinal inflammation. Prolonged use is not advised.

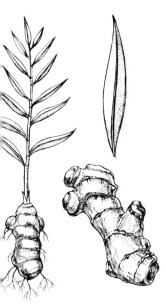

Ginger (*Zingiber officinal*)
Constituents: Volatile oil, phenols, shagaol
Ginger is a strong vasodilator and circulatory stimulant. It is also a visceral antispasmodic, digestive and carminative. Traditionally used in horses to aid expulsion of gas from the gut and as a carminative; also mixed with aloes and other purgatives to prevent griping. It is a warming agent.

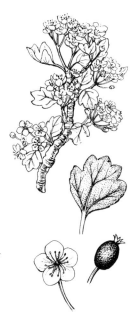

Hawthorn (*Crataegus oxyacantha*)
Constituents: Flavonoid glycosides, saponins, procyanidines, trimethyamine, condensed tannins
Used for the heart and circulation. The flavonoids dilate the coronary and peripheral arteries, and the procyanidines appear to slow the heart beat. The herb is unusual in that it has the ability both to lower blood pressure and to restore low blood pressure to normal.

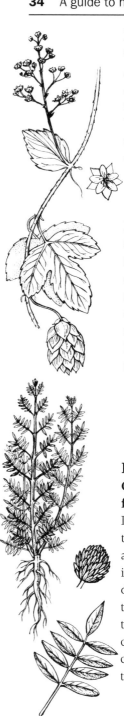

Hops (*Humulus lupulus*)
Constituents: Volatile oil, bitter resins, tannins
A valuable visceral antispasmodic and bitter tonic.
An excellent appetite stimulant and traditionally
used for its sedative action on the nervous system.
Useful in the treatment of convalescent animals, for
example after illnesses such as equine influenza,
or for problems of excitability and anxiety.

Indian hemp (*Cannabis sativa*)
Constituents: tetrahydrocannibols
Indian hemp has a powerful
effect on the central nervous
system. Traditionally used in
equine veterinary practice to
deaden pain and induce sleep.
Its use may be subject to
statutory control.

Licorice (*Glycyrrhiza glabra*)
**Constituents: Glycoside, tryterpenoid saponins,
flavonoids**
Licorice is widely used in herbal remedies. It has
the ability to harmonise with many other herbs
and its taste is not unpleasant to most horses. In
itself it is a valuable medicine mainly used for
digestive and respiratory problems. It should be
taken into account that licorice has been linked
to a rise in blood pressure in some
circumstances. It can be useful to aid a horse
coming off prolonged steroid or phenylbutazone
treatment.

Linseed (*Linum usitatissimum*)
Constituents: Mucilage, wax, glycosides

Useful in the treatment of chronic or acute
constipation. It also makes an excellent poultice
for burns when mixed with slippery elm powder.
Traditionally used as an alterative for unthrifty
horses; and given with other herbs after an illness
such as influenza or strangles.
It was often used in home-
prepared rations to provide
protein and oils to supplement
a horse's diet and improve the coat.

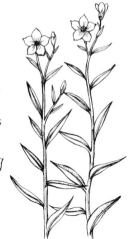

Marigold (*Calendula officinalis*)
Constituents: Carotenoids, flavonoids, bitter principle

Marigold is useful for digestive problems, and it also has important
antifungal, antibacterial and other properties. It has healing properties and can be used in the treatment of both internal and external
wounds or ulcers. It is in the same family of herbs as *Arnica*.

Meadowsweet (*Filipendula ulmaria*)
**Constituents: Salicylates, tannin, mucilage,
flavonoids, volatile oil**

Salicylic acid from meadowsweet, as well
as from willow, is the origin of aspirin.
The whole plant can be more safely
used than the isolated salicylates,
however, as the tannin and
mucilage act as a buffer,
reducing the potential for side
effects. It is a valuable anti-
inflammatory.

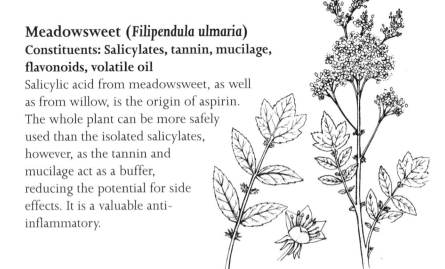

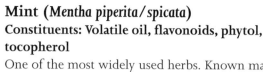

Mint (*Mentha piperita/spicata*)
Constituents: Volatile oil, flavonoids, phytol, tocopherol

One of the most widely used herbs. Known mainly for its digestive qualities, it has an antispasmodic effect on the digestive system, and may aid the expulsion of gas from the stomach or bowel. It may be used in sensible amounts as a regular addition to feed, and is useful where the horse may be prone to colic. The oil is used externally for a variety of purposes where a cooling and anaesthetic effect is required.

Nettle (*Urtica dioica*)
Constituents: Formic acid, silica, tannins

Nettle is a valuable addition to the daily diet, being rich in minerals, particularly iron, calcium and potassium. The plant helps in the absorption of iron, making it useful in the veterinary treatment of anaemia. Traditionally used as a spring tonic, it is also used in the treatment of skin ailments, such as sweet itch and other problems where a cleansing of the system is required, having great eliminative properties via the liver and kidney.

Oak bark (*Quercus robur*)
Constituents: Tannins

Oak bark is a powerful astringent, and most useful in the treatment of diarrhoea. The bark of young trees and smaller branches are the most potent source of tannin, together with the 'galls' or nut-galls. Powdered nut-galls can be used in the treatment of surface tissue, where limited circulatory effect is required. Large quantities can damage the kidneys and it should only be used under veterinary supervison.

Opium
See Poppy

Poppy (*Papaver somniferum*)
Constituents: Alkaloids (codeine, papaverine), meconic acid

Opium was once described as the 'sheet anchor of the veterinarian'. The unripe seed capsules of the opium poppy are used in the manufacture of morphine and codeine, and tincture of opium produces laudanum. Externally tincture and extract may be used to soothe pain; when used in combination with other medicines it is effective in joint and tendon injuries. Internally it can be used to control pain, and as a purgative, as well as for other uses. Its use may be subject to statutory control.

Quinine
See Cinchona

Rosehips (*Rosa rugosa, R. canina*)
Constituents: Ascorbic acid, flavonoids, tannin, mucilage

Rosehips are a rich source of natural biotin. They may be fed on a regular basis to promote healthy hoof growth. In common with all nutrients which are provided as part of the whole plant, biotin in this form is far superior to any purified source.

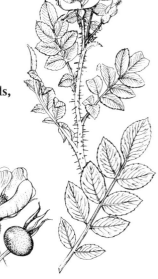

Slippery elm (*Ulmus fulva*)
Constituents: Mucilage, starch, tannin
The inner bark of the slippery elm is one of the best soothing remedies for inflammation. It lubricates and relieves gastro-intestinal irritation, and is good for diarrhoea. Externally it is useful in poultices as a healing agent for wounds.

Strophanthus (*Strophanthus hispidus*)
Constituents: Strophanthidin
Strophanthus is extremely toxic and similar in action to digitalis. It should only be used by suitably qualified veterinarians. Used in traditional veterinary medicine as an alternative to digitalis, it is more readily absorbed, and the effects on the body are not so enduring.

Valerian (*Valeriana officinalis*)
Constituents: Borneol, glycosides, isovalerianic acids, sesquiterpenes
Valerian is a potent sedative and is regularly found in mixtures which are sold to calm horses. It can also be used medically, together with other herbs, for calming digestive upsets caused by nervous tension. Valerian should not be used on a regular basis without properly qualified veterinary advice.

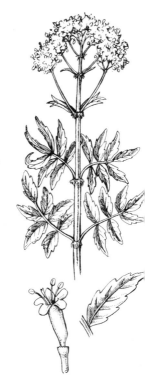

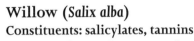

Willow (*Salix alba*)
Constituents: salicylates, tannins
The bark of the willow tree is the source of salicin, which is also contained in the bark of the poplar tree and the flower buds of meadowsweet. It is used as an anti-inflammatory and analgesic. Aspirin, which is a chemical transformation of salicin, was developed in 1876. It is now one of the most widely used drugs. Its use may contravene the rules of equestrian sport.

Witch hazel (*Hamamelis virginiana*)
Constituents: Tannin, saponins, flavonoids
The medical uses of witch hazel include the treatment of bruises and bleeding. It is traditionally used to arrest bleeding from wounds, and given for haemorrhage from the lungs and abdominal organs. Also used in the treatment of piles in foals.

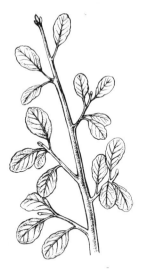

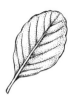

9 Herbal medicine and the law

There is no recognised training or qualification for veterinary herbalists, as there is for those practising in human herbal medicine. Even if there were, the Veterinary Surgeons Act prohibits, anyone who is not a veterinary surgeon to treat or give advice for the treatment of any condition or disease of an animal. There are no exceptions to this rule; the Act is quite clear and unequivocal.

Veterinary surgeons will indicate their membership of the Royal College with the letters MRCVS or FRCVS after their name. Generally speaking those who do not do so are not veterinary surgeons and should not be consulted. The same applies to homoeopathy and acupuncture.

Those qualified in allied subjects such as nutrition, acupuncture, chiropractic or physiotherapy, can only practice if they are under the direct supervision of a veterinary surgeon at all times. If acting alone they must not treat or give advice. Owners seeking help from those who are not veterinary surgeons are liable to prosecution under Animal Welfare legislation if allowing, or seeking, such help causes an increase in or fails to alleviate suffering and pain.

10 British Association of Holistic Nutrition and Medicine

Holistic feeding stuffs and supplements

Holistic practices and principles in nutrition and medicine were defined according to the scientific theory of holism, first published by Jan Christian Smuts.

Equine feeding stuffs and supplements licensed by the BAHNM as holistic products can be identified by a symbol which is carried on all packaging. Manufacturers must satisfy the BAHNM Certification Committee that the product complies with holistic protocols and satisfies regulations in the primary areas of safety, efficacy and quality.

The BAHNM takes advice from its own scientific and legal advisers and also works with government departments involved with relevant legislation, such as the Feeding Stuffs Regulations, the Medicines Act and the Trade Descriptions Act.

The Association provides independent and impartial information

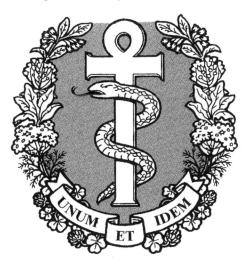

The symbol of the British Association of Holistic Nutrition and Medicine which is carried on the packaging of licensed products.

and advice in technical material and reference books, as well as a telephone helpline for information on the following:

Health issues raised by inappropriate use of raw materials in feeding stuffs and supplements

Consumer rights

The Feeding Stuffs Regulations

The BAHNM Regulations

Licensed holistic feeding stuffs and supplements

The Medicines Act

Licensed medicinal products

The Veterinary Surgeons Act and the law concerning the treatment of animals

11 The Medicines Act

Medical products

Any product sold to be given to the horse by mouth should be covered by the Feeding Stuffs Regulations or the Medicines Act. Which legislation applies depends mainly on the claims being made for the product. The legal definition is that if a 'medical claim' is made for the product it comes under the Medicines Act, but if there is no medical claim it comes under the Feeding Stuffs Regulations.

If a product comes under the Medicines Act, it must have a licence issued through the Veterinary Medicines Directorate. The product must satisfy conditions in the primary areas of safety, quality, and efficacy.

Because many feed supplements are not officially recognised as medicinal products they automatically come under the Feeding Stuffs Regulations. This means that the ingredients can be expressed in a way which conceals their exact nature. The BAHNM can advise the consumer in these circumstances.

12 The Trading Standards Department

The Trading Standards Department's duties are to improve and maintain standards of fair trading in terms of quality, quantity, safety and description.

The department carries out its duties through inspection, sampling, testing and investigation. It will enforce legislation by prosecution if necessary.

It also informs, advises and educates manufacturers, traders and consumers. The department works closely with government departments as well as outside bodies.

The department gives free, impartial and strictly confidential advice. There is never any reference made to the name of any individual making a complaint.

Glossary of terms used to describe the actions of herbs when used in a remedy

Abortifacient Causes abortion – premature expulsion of foetus

Adaptogenic Helps to restore balance within the body

Alterative Produces gradually beneficial effects through detoxification and improving nutrition

Anaesthetic Deadens sensation and reduces pain

Analgesic Pain relieving

Anodyne Pain relieving

Antacid Reduces stomach acid

Anthelmintic Destroys or expels intestinal worms

Anti-allergic Reduces the effects of allergic reactions

Anti-anaemic Treats anaemia

Antibacterial Destroys or stops the growth of bacterial infections

Antibiotic Destroys or stops the growth of bacteria

Antimucous/catarrhal Reduces mucus/catarrh

Antidepressant Relieves symptoms of depression

Anti-emetic Relieves nausea and vomiting

Antifungal Treats fungal infections

Antihaemorrhagic Stops bleeding and haemorrhage

Antihistamine Neutralises the effects of histamine in an allergic response

Antihydrotic Reduces or suppresses perspiration

Anti-inflammatory Reduces inflammation

Antilithic Dissolves stones or gravel in the kidneys or bladder

Antimicrobial Destroys or stops the growth of micro-organisms

Antineoplastic Has anti-cancer properties

Antirheumatic Relieves rheumatism/arthritis

Antiseptic Prevents putrefaction

Antispasmodic Prevents or relieves spasms or cramps

Antithrombotic Prevents blood clots

Antitoxic Clears toxins from the system

Antitussive Relieves coughing

Antiviral Destroys or stops the growth of viral infections

Astringent Contracts tissue, reducing secretions or discharges

Bitter Increases appetite and promotes digestion

Carminative Eases cramping pains and expels flatulence

Cell proliferator Enhances the formation of new tissue to speed the healing process

* From A. McIntyre, *Herbs for common ailments* (Gaia, 1992)

Cholagogue Increases flow of bile into the intestines

Convalescent Speeds recovery during convalescence

Demulcent Soothes irritated tissues, especially mucous membrane

Depurative Cleanses and purifies the system, especially the blood

Diaphoretic Promotes perspiration

Digestive Aids digestion

Diuretic Promotes the flow of urine

Emetic Causes vomiting

Emmenagogue Promotes menstrual flow (avoid in pregnancy)

Emollient Soothes and heals the skin

Expectorant Promotes expulsion of mucus from the respiratory tract

Febrifuge Reduces fever

Galactagogue Increases milk flow

Haemostatic Stops bleeding and haemorrhage

Hormone balancer Improves hormone balance

Hypnotic Induces sleep

Hypoglycaemic Reduces blood sugar

Hypotensive Reduces blood pressure

Immune enhancer Helps the functioning of the immune system

Laxative Promotes evacuation of the bowels

Narcotic Relieves pain and induces sleep

Nervine Calms the nerves

Nutritive Contains nutritious substances

Oestrogenic Resembles the actions of oestrogen

Oxytocic Stimulates contraction of uterine muscle and so facilitates childbirth

Parasiticide Kills parasites

Parturient Facilitates childbirth

Partus praeparator Prepares for childbirth

Purgative Produces vigorous emptying of the bowels

Relaxant Relaxes nerves and muscles

Restorative Restores normal physiological activity

Rubefacient A gentle local irritation that produces redness of the skin

Sedative Reduces nervousness and anxiety, induces sleep

Stimulant Produces energy

Stomachic Stimulates, strengthens, or tones the stomach

Styptic Stems bleeding

Sudorific Promotes perspiration

Tonic Invigorates and tones the body and promotes wellbeing

Vasodilator Widens blood vessels, lowering blood pressure

Vulnerary Promotes wound healing

Useful addresses

ADAS (Food Farming, Land and Leisure), *see local directories*

British Association of Holistic Nutrition and Medicine, 8 Borough Court Road, Hartley Wintney, Basingstoke, Hants RG27 8JA. Helpline tel. 01252 843282

British Association of Homoeopathic Veterinary Surgeons, Alternative Veterinary Medicine Centre, Chinham House, Stanford in the Vale, Faringdon, Oxon SN7 8NQ

British Veterinary Association, 7 Mansfield Street, London W1M 0AT

Ministry of Agriculture, Fisheries and Food, Ergon House, % Nobel House, 17 Smith Square, London SW1P 3JR. Tel. 0171 238 3000

Royal College of Veterinary Surgeons, 32 Belgrave Square, London SW1 8QP. Tel. 0171 222 2001 (Membership)

Trading Standards Department, *see local directories*

Veterinary Medicines Directorate, Central Veterinary Laboratory, New Haw, Weybridge, Surrey KT1S 1BR. Tel. 01932 336911

British Library Cataloguing in Publication Data
A catalogue record for this book is available from the British Library.

ISBN 0.85131.646.8

Published in Great Britain in 1995 by

J. A. Allen & Company Limited
an imprint of Robert Hale Ltd.
Clerkenwell House,
45–47 Clerkenwell Green,
London, EC1R 0HT.

Reprinted 2000
Reprinted 2003

© J. A. Allen & Company Limited 1995

Typeset by Textype Typesetters, Cambridge
Printed in Hong Kong by Midas Printing International Ltd